Affirmations
for your
Healthy
Pregnancy

Affirmative Press   1992

Cheryl Kilvington
Robert F. Brunjes

Bibliography

Columbia University College of Physicians & Surgeons Complete Guide to Pregnancy by Donald F. Tapley, MD and W. Duane Todd, MD, Crown Publishers, Inc., New York 1988.

Childbirth With Love by Dr. Niels H. Laversen, G.P. Putnam's Sons, New York 1983.

The Well Pregnancy Book by Mike Samuels & Nancy Samuels, Summit Books, New York 1986.

What to Expect When You're Expecting by Arlene Eisenberg, Heidi Eisenberg Murkoff, and Sandee Eisenberg Hathaway, R.N., Workman Publishing, New York 1988.

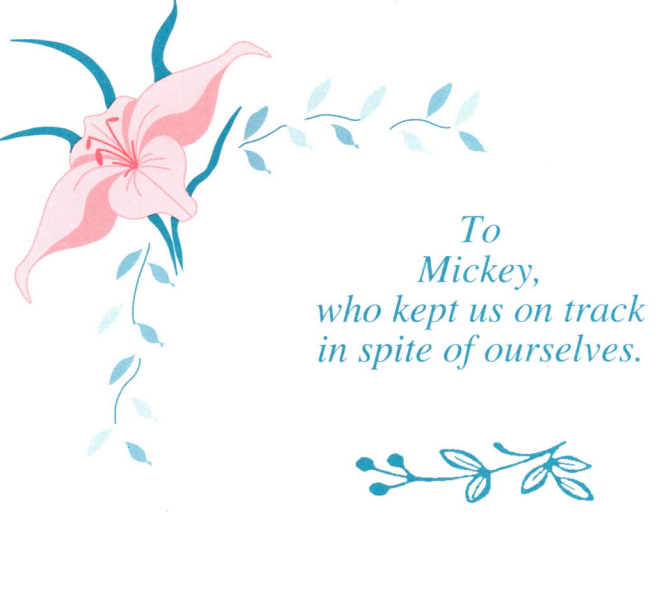

*To
Mickey,
who kept us on track
in spite of ourselves.*

Congratulations!

You are going to have a baby! This perpetual calendar, *Affirmations for your Healthy Pregnancy*, has been written just for you. It is intended to keep you informed of your baby's growth and development every day of your pregnancy and to help you lovingly affirm to your baby the wonder and perfection of its existence in our world.

Each baby is an individual and experiences its growth and development on its own individual timetable; therefore the developmental stages you read about on these pages are approximations based on average fetal development. Your baby's actual development may vary from the information contained on these pages.

This perpetual calendar is intended to enhance the experience of your pregnancy. It is not intended to replace prenatal medical care, proper nutrition or exercise.

Dearest baby,
it is safe and loving here
in our world; we welcome
you with open arms.

Week Forty-two: Saturday

About 5% of all deliveries are *postterm*, or take place
between the 42nd and 44th weeks of the pregnancy.

Dating your pregnancy . . .

The fetal development information contained on these pages begins with the moment of conception. Because the actual date of conception can only be guessed at, medical personnel date the pregnancy from the beginning of the mother's last period, although conception generally takes place about two weeks later. Thus a pregnancy dated by your doctor at 20 weeks gestation is actually 18 weeks *postconception*. Likewise, it is often stated that most babies are delivered at about 40 weeks, which is actually 38 weeks *postconception*. To coincide with the dating used by your doctor, this calendar begins at week three, which is the *first week following actual conception.*

To begin using this calendar . . . count the weeks that have elapsed since the first day of your last period. Find that week in this calendar, turn to the present day of the week, and begin affirming your healthy pregnancy.

I actively seek to be relaxed and happy, sweet child, and to lovingly remain in control of your birth.

Week Forty-two: Friday

Studies have shown that women who enter labor with a positive relaxed attitude have less pain, and contractions proceed steadily and effectively.

We are lovingly creating a healthy beautiful baby.

Week Three: Sunday

The egg that will become your baby is fertilized with its father's sperm.

Darling baby, you are encouraged to choose your time of birth whenever you are ready.

Week Forty-two: Thursday

Some medical theories based on animal research attribute the onset of labor to hormones released by the baby itself.

Sweet child,
we are giving you the
best of ourselves.

The egg accepts the sperm and becomes fertilized.

Welcome, little baby!
We welcome you to come
into our world at any time.

Week Forty-two: Wednesday

The mother experiences a blood-tinged mucous discharge when her mucous plug slips out of the cervix, signaling the onset of labor by hours to days.

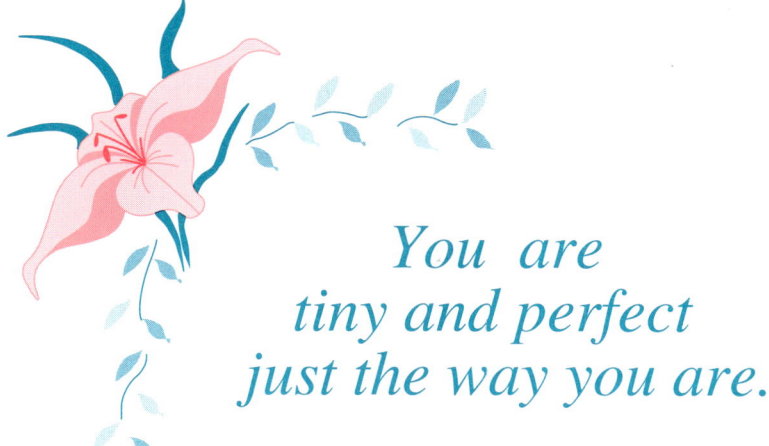

You are
tiny and perfect
just the way you are.

Week Three: Tuesday

The tiny fertilized egg begins to divide into a cluster of many smaller cells.

*I gladly accept
these new conditions,
sweet child, because I
know you are almost ready
to be born!*

Week Forty-two: Tuesday

Lightening eases the mother's breathing and adds to the frequency of urination, low backache, and leg swelling.

*You are having
a safe and healthy journey,
my little darling.*

Week Three: Wednesday

The egg travels down the mother's Fallopian tube.

Dear baby,
I love you so much and
can't wait to hold you
in my arms.

Week Forty-two: Monday

First time mothers may experience lightening two to three weeks prior to birth; subsequent pregnancies experience lightening shortly before labor begins.

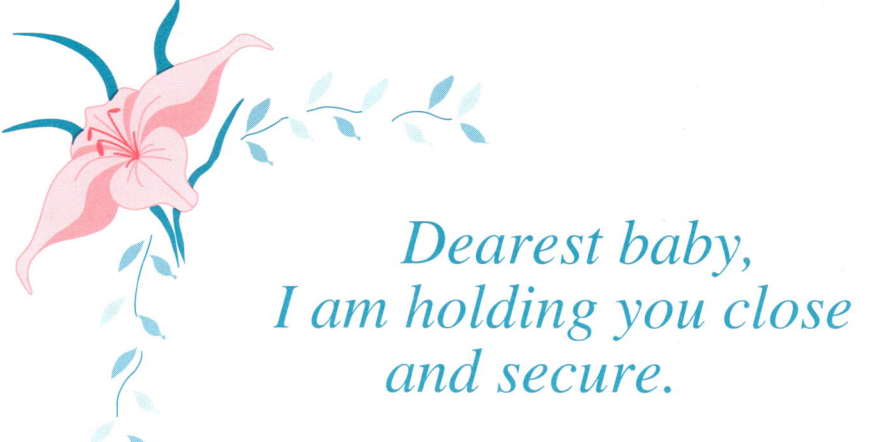

Dearest baby,
I am holding you close
and secure.

Week Three: Thursday

The fertilized egg attaches itself to the endometrial
lining of the mother's uterus.

*Precious infant,
you are in the perfect
position for a gentle, easy
entrance to the world.*

Week Forty-two: Sunday

Lightening or *dropping* refers to the baby dropping down into the pelvis, signaling the approach of birth.

Welcome,
sweet baby! I welcome
you with an open heart.

Week Three: Friday

The mother experiences natural changes in her
immune system that prevent her body from rejecting
this new tissue.

Both of us are prepared for your final journey into waiting loving arms, sweet baby.

Week Forty-one: Saturday

Effacing (shortening) and *dilating* (widening) of the cervix is a process called *ripening*, indicating that the cervix is ready for labor.

Make yourself comfortable, little darling. You are a beautiful healthy creation of love.

Week Three: Saturday

The fertilized egg continues cell division as it implants more firmly in the mother's womb.

Dearest child,
your journey into our
world will be easy
and natural.

Week Forty-one: Friday

Imperceptible prelabor contractions during the ninth
month of pregnancy soften the cervix before labor.

*My blood is healthy
and abundant, little one.
Use as much as you need
to grow big and strong.*

Week Four: Sunday

The embryo begins to extract blood from the interuterine lining of the mother.

Everything is happening on schedule, little one, so that you can join us safely and easily.

Week Forty-one: Thursday

The lower part of the uterus begins to stretch, preparing the cervix to open so your baby can emerge.

Sweet baby,
I give you all the love
and nourishment you need.

Week Four: Monday

Nutrients are supplied to your developing baby from its mother's uterus.

*My body is
guiding you down the path
to a whole new world,
darling baby.*

During these last few weeks, the upper part of the uterus has stopped expanding and started to contract in preparation for labor.

Dear baby,
you are strong and healthy
and beautiful.

Week Four: Tuesday

Your baby's cells continue to divide rapidly.

Sweet baby, our world welcomes your presence and invites you to join us.

Week Forty-one: Tuesday

The exact cause of the onset of labor is unknown, but the size of your baby and its maturity may have an effect on the length of your pregnancy.

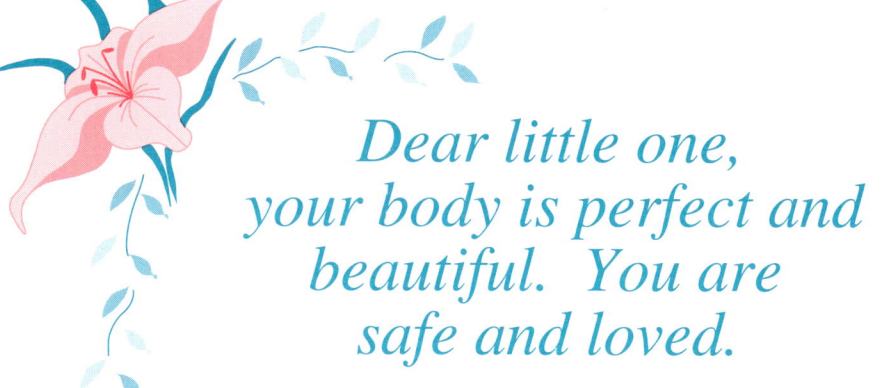

Dear little one,
your body is perfect and
beautiful. You are
safe and loved.

Week Four: Wednesday

The rapidly dividing cells of your baby begin to
cluster according to their future functions.

*Dearest infant,
whenever you are ready to
join us, we are ready and
excited to hold you close.*

<u>*Week Forty-one: Monday*</u>

Few babies (about 5%) actually arrive on the day they
are expected.

Sweet baby, you are growing and developing perfectly! My love keeps you safe and warm.

Week Four: Thursday

Your baby's cell clusters become postured for eventual organ development.

Darling baby,
we welcome your
appearance and bid you
enter our world.

Week Forty-one: Sunday

Birth is expected some time within the 40th week, although any time between the 38th and 42nd weeks is quite common.

*I send you lots of
love and nourishment,
little baby. Your body is
growing strong and healthy.*

Week Four: Friday

Groups of cells are preparing to develop into your baby's body systems.

You are the perfect size, little one; you are perfectly healthy and ready to fill our waiting arms.

Week Forty: Saturday

Your baby is probably close to 20 inches long.

*Everything works
perfectly, sweet baby.
You are loved and nourished.
Grow strong!*

Week Four: Saturday

Cell division continues as your baby selectively
groups cells into eventual functions.

You are the
perfect weight for who
you are, darling child.

Your baby's weight varies widely from five to ten pounds.

*I send you lots of love
and nourishment, little baby.
Your body is growing
strong and healthy.*

Week Five: Sunday

Your baby is forming a distinct head and tail fold.

Sweet child, you are protected and safe from everything. We welcome you with love.

Week Forty: Thursday

Creamy white vernix still covers your baby's body except for its mouth and eyes.

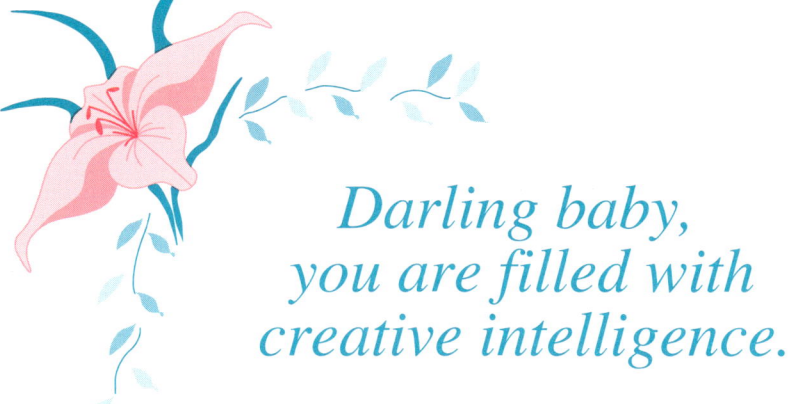

Darling baby,
you are filled with
creative intelligence.

Week Five: Monday

The brain of your baby begins to develop.

*Your hair is shiny
and healthy, dear baby;
your beautiful hair is a
sign of your individuality.*

Your baby's scalp hair varies from 0 - 1 1/2 inches long.

Dear little one,
your mommy sends you
lots of love from her heart
to yours.

Week Five: Tuesday

Your baby begins to form its heart, which at this stage is a single tube.

Your skin is strong and beautiful, little one, and you are ready to make your debut!

Week Forty: Tuesday

Most of the downy fuzz on your baby's body has disappeared.

Your loving heart
works perfectly, sweet baby.
Fill your heart with love!

Week Five: Wednesday

Your baby's simple heart begins the contraction process.

*You are healthy
and plump and cute as
a button, little baby.*

Week Forty: Monday

Your baby's body has filled out and its appearance is
round and plump.

*Your blood is filled
with joy, sweet child, moving
through every part of you.
Feel joyful!*

Week Five: Thursday

As your baby's heart contracts, it forces blood through the embryo and placenta.

Sweet baby,
your beautiful, protective
skin is ready to face
the world.

Week Forty: Sunday

Your baby's skin is pretty and smooth.

Your blood is moving through you, little darling, bringing all the love and nourishment you need.

Week Five: Friday

Your baby is developing a primitive circulatory system.

*My darling child,
your perception and
sensitivity are a miracle.*

Week Thirty-nine: Saturday

Your baby's responses to its mother's emotions have become quite sophisticated; its heart rate can increase as its mother contemplates eating a sweet dessert!

Every part of you is absolutely perfect, my sweet baby. You are continuing to grow healthy and strong.

<u>*Week Five: Saturday*</u>

Your baby's organs are beginning to develop.

Sweet baby,
my activities and yours
are in continuous
loving interaction.

Week Thirty-nine: Friday

Increased blood sugar in the mother makes your baby's movements more noticeable after a meal.

My darling child,
each side of you is
beautiful and perfect.
I love you.

Week Six: Sunday

Paired cells align themselves along each side of your baby to form the two symmetrical halves of its body.

Dearest infant,
we welcome the miracle
of watching your beautiful
eyes take on their final hue!

Week Thirty-nine: Thursday

The iris of your baby's eyes remains slate blue until after birth.

*Life is full of wonder,
sweet baby, and you are
digesting it all!*

Week Six: Monday

Your baby's digestive tract begins to form.

*Every tiny detail
of your development is
perfect, little one; we
welcome you with lots of love.*

Week Thirty-nine: Wednesday

The whites of your baby's eyes have turned fairly white in color.

*Look with eyes
of wonder, little darling,
at the perfection
of your world.*

Week Six: Tuesday

The eyes of your baby are beginning to develop.

*Sweet baby, you are
loved because you are you;
we welcome the gender you
have chosen for yourself.*

Week Thirty-nine: Tuesday

Female genitalia is completely developed; testicles of
most male babies have descended into the scrotum.

Sweet child,
your heart is strong and
full of love and joy.

Week Six: Wednesday

Your baby's heart is now beating rhythmically.

Stand on your tiptoes and reach for your dreams, dearest baby!

Week Thirty-nine: Monday

Your baby's toenails have reached the ends of its toes.

*I lovingly give
to you all that you need
right now, my darling child.*

Week Six: Thursday

You and your baby are continually exchanging oxygen, carbon dioxide, and nutrients.

You are perfect right down to your tiny fingernails, sweet child.

Week Thirty-nine: Sunday

Your baby's fingernails have now grown beyond the ends of its fingertips.

Sweet baby,
your world is filled with
beautiful sounds to
hear and explore.

Week Six: Friday

The ears of your baby are starting to form.

I sense your breathing movements, little one, and congratulate you for your loving trust and acceptance of life.

Week Thirty-eight: Saturday

In some mothers, the abdomen may visibly rise and fall with the rapid rhythmic movements of the baby's chest wall.

*You are tiny
and perfect, little one,
and growing more beautiful
each day.*

Week Six: Saturday

Your baby is now 1/4 inch long.

*You are breathing
in life, sweet baby, as
surely as you will breathe
the air when you are born.*

Week Thirty-eight: Friday

Your baby establishes spontaneous breathing movements, even though its lungs will not be fully inflated until the baby is outside the womb.

*Breathe in life,
sweet baby! Life is our
most precious gift.*

Week Seven: Sunday

Your baby's lungs are in the process of forming.

"Sweet little baby, don't you cry, Mama's gonna sing you a lullaby..."

Week Thirty-eight: Thursday

Research has shown that your unborn baby often responds to its mother's voice by moving in rhythm to it.

*Reach out
and grasp the wonder
of your new life,
little darling.*

Week Seven: Monday

Tiny buds of arms and legs appear on your baby.

Your world is gentle and loving, darling baby. You are safe and secure.

Week Thirty-eight: Wednesday

Parents can rub the mother's abdomen gently and talk soothingly to quiet their startled baby.

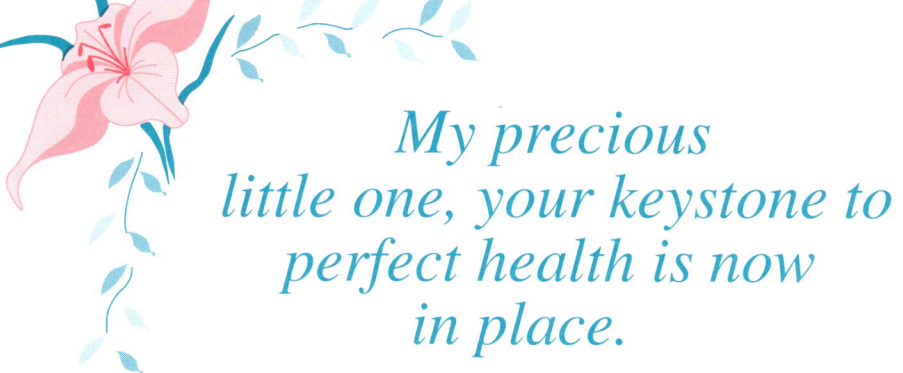

*My precious
little one, your keystone to
perfect health is now
in place.*

Week Seven: Tuesday

Your baby's liver is beginning to develop.

*Your growth
is remarkable, sweet child;
you are big and strong
and healthy.*

Week Thirty-eight: Tuesday

Your baby is over 18 inches long and weighs over six pounds.

Sweet baby,
every part of your brain
is bright and capable.

Regional divisions form in your baby's brain.

We are healthy and comfortable, little baby, as we look forward to your entrance into this wonderful world.

Week Thirty-eight: Monday

After engagement, the mother usually feels more comfortable because there is less pressure on her lungs and stomach.

Darling child,
you have everything you
need right now.
You are perfect!

Week Seven: Thursday

A primitive set of temporary kidneys are forming for your baby.

Sweet baby,
you are moving into place
perfectly as we prepare
for your birth.

Week Thirty-eight: Sunday

Your baby's head moves down into the mother's pelvis and becomes *engaged*.

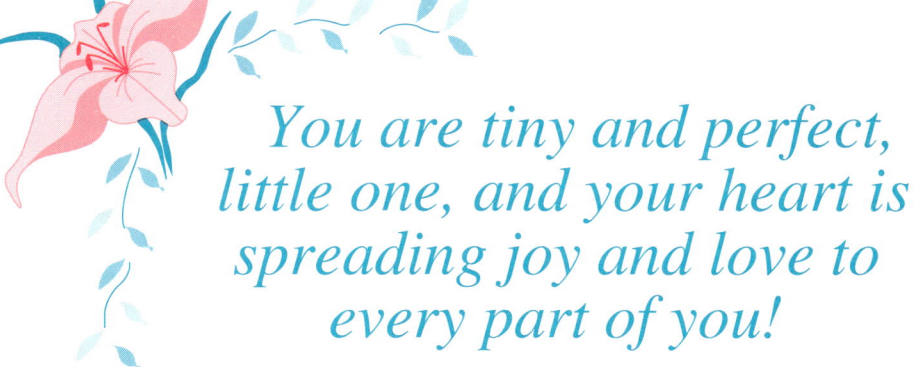

You are tiny and perfect, little one, and your heart is spreading joy and love to every part of you!

Week Seven: Friday

Your baby's heart pushes newly formed blood around its pea-sized body.

I send you plenty of nourishing blood to suppy your needs, my darling child.

Week Thirty-seven: Saturday

To reduce leg swelling and varicose veins, it is advisable for the mother to lie on her side rather than her back; this allows her heart to increase its output by about 22%.

Precious baby,
you are balanced and
centered; your perfect little
body provides everything
you need.

Week Seven: Saturday

Hormones from the placenta take the place of the mother's hormones.

*I lovingly
make room for you,
sweet baby, in my body
and in our family.*

Week Thirty-seven: Friday

During pregnancy, the mother's uterus grows from 500 to 1000 times its nonpregnant size to accommodate her growing baby.

*Grow,
my little darling!
You are growing and
forming beautifully!*

Week Eight: Sunday

Your baby has grown to one inch long, 1/3 of which
is its head.

Everything develops in the perfect time and sequence, little one; you are perfect in every way.

Week Thirty-seven: Thursday

Your baby's various vital organs continue to develop and mature.

My precious little one, you have everything you need to be supported in life!

<u>*Week Eight: Monday*</u>

The main internal organs have finished forming within your baby's body.

*I hold you close
to my heart, little sweetheart,
and I anticipate holding
you in my arms.*

Week Thirty-seven: Wednesday

Your baby is in a head down position, ready for birth.

Your heart is strong and full of love, sweet baby. Love and joy are spreading throughout your body.

Week Eight: Tuesday

Your baby's strongly beating heart has fused into four chambers and its circulatory system is well established.

*Your liver is your key
to good health, sweet baby,
and it is developing perfectly.*

Week Thirty-seven: Tuesday

Your baby's liver is still immature and developing prior to birth.

Sweet baby,
your world is safe
and full of wonder
to feel, hear, and see.

Week Eight: Wednesday

The reflexes are present and your baby is responsive to touch, sound, and light.

Dearest baby,
we are both feeling limited
in our movements, but we are
together sharing space and
life and love!

Week Thirty-seven: Monday

The baby's mother generally feels very heavy and
uncomfortable at this time.

Reach out,
little one, and accept
all the love and joy
your world has to offer you.

Week Eight: Thursday

Paddles have developed at the ends of your baby's arms.

Darling child,
I caress you gently through
my skin and cherish you
as you grow and mature.

Week Thirty-seven: Sunday

Your baby now fills the uterus and it cannot move
around freely.

Your body
is your world to touch
and explore, little darling.

Week Eight: Friday

Your baby can touch parts of its body with its hands
and feet as well as with the umbilical cord.

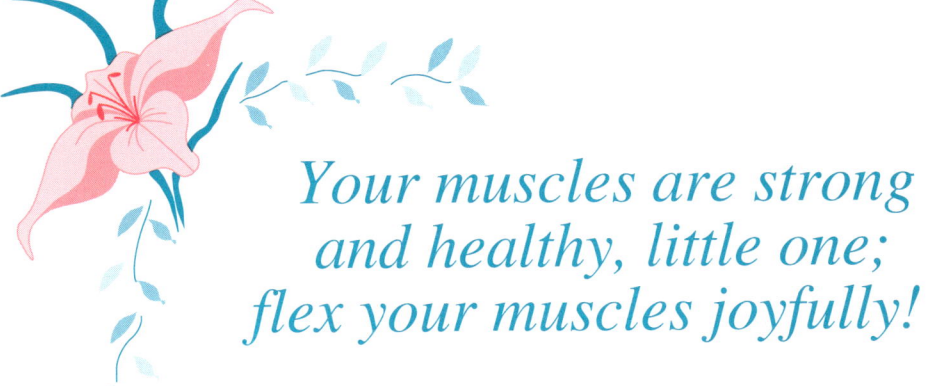

Your muscles are strong and healthy, little one; flex your muscles joyfully!

Week Thirty-six: Saturday

Your baby's muscle tone continues to improve.

Trust in your own responses, darling child; your perceptions are perfect for you right now.

Week Eight: Saturday

Currently, your baby will move away from things that touch it, but later in development will move toward them.

*Life flows in and out
of your lungs with perfect
ease, sweet child; you have
the power to take in life fully.*

Week Thirty-six: Friday

Your baby's lungs are now fully developed.

Reach out your hands,
my sweet little one,
and grasp the excitement
of life!

Week Nine: Sunday

Your baby's hands have completely formed, although refinements will continue for some time.

*Dance on the tips
of your sweet toes,
darling baby; we have lots
of cause for celebration!*

Week Thirty-six: Thursday

Your baby's toenails are still moving toward the tips of its toes.

Darling baby,
I love you in more ways
than your precious
fingers can count.

Week Nine: Monday

Fingers are now beginning to separate on your baby's hands.

*Your beautiful
hands are there to reach
out and grasp the wonder
of life, sweet child.*

Week Thirty-six: Wednesday

The nails on your baby's hands have reached the
fingertips.

*Your darling
little feet will carry you
off to a life of love
and adventure.*

Week Nine: Tuesday

The feet of your baby have formed and the beginnings of toes are evident.

You are growing so beautifully, little sweetheart; you are perfect in every way.

Week Thirty-six: Tuesday

Your baby is now 17-18 inches long and weighs about 5 1/2 pounds.

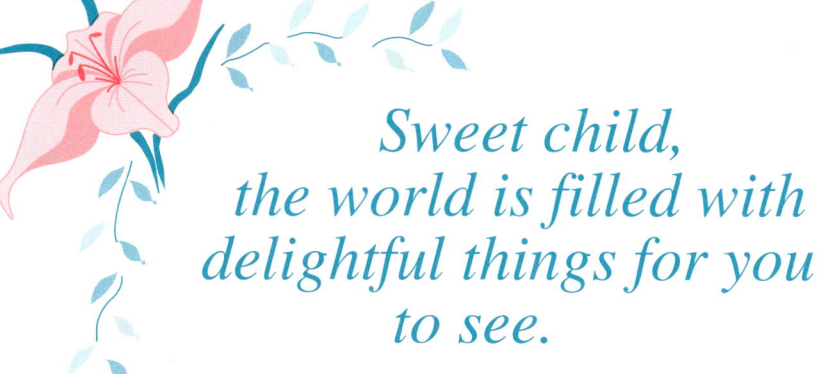

Sweet child,
the world is filled with
delightful things for you
to see.

Week Nine: Wednesday

Eyelids are forming over your baby's eyes.

*We release and let go
of all we no longer need,
darling baby; it is safe to
let go and welcome the new.*

Week Thirty-six: Monday

Your baby's kidneys are now fully mature.

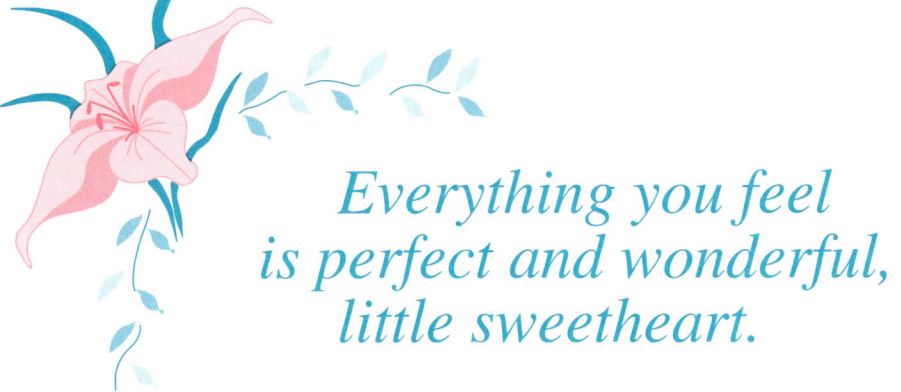

Everything you feel
is perfect and wonderful,
little sweetheart.

Week Nine: Thursday

Your baby's nervous system continues to develop.

Sweet child,
we breathe in life and love
as we continue down the
path toward your birth.

Week Thirty-six: Sunday

Raising the arms overhead lifts the mother's ribcage
and gives her lungs more space.

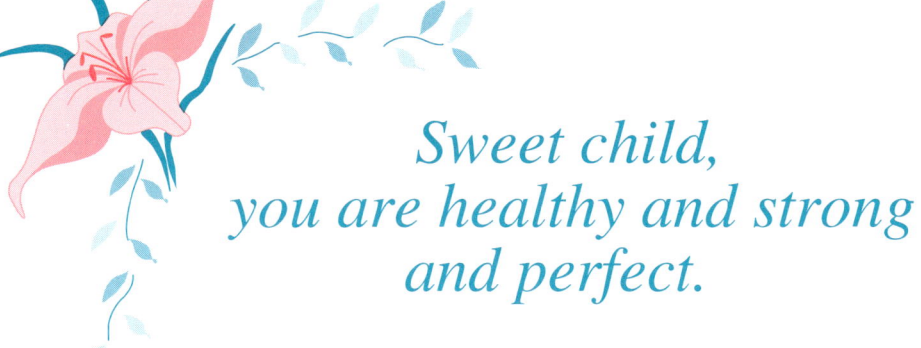

Sweet child,
you are healthy and strong
and perfect.

Week Nine: Friday

Muscle fiber begins to develop in your baby's body.

*Darling child,
we both have all the precious
air we need; life supports us
in our journey together.*

Week Thirty-five: Saturday

As the pregnancy progresses, the uterus pushes up the mother's diaphragm, giving a feeling of less room to breathe.

*Your perfect
little body has everything
you need, little one.*

Your baby's tail disappears as its body develops.

*Together we
enjoy our gentle exercise,
sweet baby; we are lovingly
enhancing your strength
and health.*

Week Thirty-five: Friday

Regular gentle exercise and elevating the legs can lessen the incidence of muscle spasms in the mother's legs.

Sweet baby,
you are growing so big
and strong and lovable!

Week Ten: Sunday

Your baby has grown to 1 1/2 inches long.

Darling baby,
your presence in my life
is worth far more than
any discomfort. I love you!

Week Thirty-five: Thursday

Increased pressure from the uterus on nerves and
veins can cause leg cramps for the mother.

Dearest little infant,
you are becoming your
own person and we love
who you are.

Week Ten: Monday

Facial features on your baby are recognizable.

You are developing perfectly, little one; life supports us just as we are.

<u>*Week Thirty-five: Wednesday*</u>

Your baby's head and body have reached the same proportion they will be at birth.

You have everything you need, sweetheart, to draw in nourishment and love.

Week Ten: Tuesday

Ten tooth buds make their first appearance in your baby's mouth.

Breathe in life,
sweet child! You are a
most deserving
child of life.

Week Thirty-five: Tuesday

Your baby's lungs have developed to almost full
maturity.

*Your body
is forming perfectly,
little baby; you are strong
and healthy.*

Week Ten: Wednesday

The cartilage of your baby's pre-skeleton forms.

*Your skin is
healthy and smooth,
precious baby; your beautiful
skin is an expression of your
individuality.*

Week Thirty-five: Monday

Most of your baby's skin wrinkles have disappeared
with the accumulation of more fat cells.

*Dance to the music
of life, sweet baby,
you have lots of room
to move!*

Week Ten: Thursday

Your baby begins to move its arms and legs.

*All of your needs
are fulfilled, little one;
you are becoming more
perfect each day.*

Week Thirty-five: Sunday

Your baby continues to gain more fat cells.

*I trust that
you are moving and
having the time of your life,
little one!*

Week Ten: Friday

Your baby's movements are, as yet, undetectable by its mother.

Darling baby,
warm milk, a warm bath,
and relaxation exercises
help me get lots of rest
for both of us.

Week Thirty-four: Saturday

Mother's sleep may be interrupted by anticipation, anxiety, fetal movements, or muscle cramps.

Your little world
is yours to explore,
sweet baby. Everything
about you is perfect.

Week Ten: Saturday

Your baby continues to touch its own body with its hands and feet.

*My muscles
are strong and limber,
little baby, and they
hold you easily.*

Week Thirty-four: Friday

Regular abdominal exercises can strengthen the muscles that support the uterus.

Sweet little child,
you are distinctly individual
and loved for who you are.

Week Eleven: Sunday

Your baby's external genitalia begin to make an appearance.

Sweet child,
I take good care of us by
maintaining good posture
and tilting my pelvis back
when I stand or walk.

Week Thirty-four: Thursday

Mother often experiences lower back pain during this time due to the forward tilting of her pelvis as her uterus enlarges.

*You are free
to be either a boy or a girl,
little love, because we
love you no matter what.*

Week Eleven: Monday

Your baby's sex is still undeterminable for several more weeks.

*You are big and
strong and healthy,
sweetheart, and growing
more each day.*

Week Thirty-four: Wednesday

Your baby is about 16 1/2 inches long and weighs
about 5 pounds.

Speak out,
sweet child! In this family
you will be free to speak
your highest truth.

Week Eleven: Tuesday

Your baby's larynx begins to form.

I feel you
moving inside of me,
sweet baby; move to your
heart's content.

Week Thirty-four: Tuesday

Your baby's increased size means there is less room
to move around; therefore movements may be felt
more strongly by the mother.

*The world is full
of incredible ideas for you
to digest, little one, and you
are free to accept or discard
what you will.*

Week Eleven: Wednesday

The digestive tract is being perfected in your baby.

I welcome your activity, little darling; you are healthy and active and bright!

Week Thirty-four: Monday

Your baby is likely to move vigorously throughout this stage of development.

Grow, sweet baby,
you are growing so big
and strong!

Your baby's body growth continues at a rapid rate.

Precious child,
make yourself warm and
comfortable and I will
cuddle you close.

Week Thirty-four: Sunday

Your baby is likely lying with its head down toward
the mother's pelvis.

Feel the loving touch of Life and enjoy those sweet sensations, dearest one.

Week Eleven: Friday

Sensitivity to touch is spreading throughout your baby's body.

Sweet baby,
you are welcome to
express yourself through
your activity.

Week Thirty-three: Saturday

The activity level of your unborn baby often indicates
how active your baby will be after birth.

*You are safe
and secure in your
little world, my child.*

Week Eleven: Saturday

Your baby's head remains relatively insensitive to touch, probably as a protection during its development.

Dream big,
sweet darling! Your dreams
will shape your world.

Week Thirty-three: Friday

Brain wave tests at this stage detect REM or rapid eye movement during sleep, indicating that your baby is capable of dreaming.

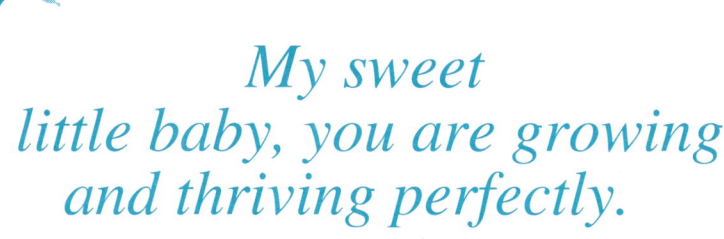

*My sweet
little baby, you are growing
and thriving perfectly.*

Week Twelve: Sunday

Your baby is now 2 1/4 inches long.

*You are welcome
to move around and play,
little one; I love to
watch you play.*

Week Thirty-three: Thursday

Your baby's fist or foot will sometimes make a
distinct bulge on its mother's tummy.

*Move and play
to your heart's content,
my precious little one.*

Week Twelve: Monday

Your baby has increased its movements within the
womb.

*I can see and feel
your movements, sweet baby;
you are free to move to
the music of life.*

Week Thirty-three: Wednesday

Your baby's vigorous movements are now visible on
the outside of its mother's abdomen.

Your hands are becoming more complete each day, sweet baby, and you are free to grasp the wonder of life.

Week Twelve: Tuesday

Your baby is beginning to form fingernails.

*Your heartbeat
is uniquely yours, my child,
a perfect expression of
your individuality.*

Week Thirty-three: Tuesday

Research shows that each human being possesses a characteristic heartbeat, which remains more or less consistant from pre-birth to old age.

*Your feet
will carry you on
wonderful adventures
in life, sweet baby.*

Week Twelve: Wednesday

Toenails are forming on your baby's feet.

*Your heart is beating
perfectly, precious baby.
Let love and joy flow
through your veins.*

Week Thirty-three: Monday

Your baby's heartbeat varies from 120 to 160 beats
per minute, about double its mother's rate.

Take in all
of life's nourishment,
sweet little baby, you are
digesting life easily.

Week Twelve: Thursday

Digestive juices are being produced by your baby's
liver.

*Fill your heart
with joy, little one, and
pump it throughout your
perfect little body.*

Week Thirty-three: Sunday

Your baby's muffled heartbeat can now be heard through the stethoscope.

*Your blood
is healthy and strong,
dear child, and flowing
easily through your body.*

Week Twelve: Friday

Your baby's liver produces red corpuscles.

Darling baby,
I fill my life with affirming
thoughts and surround us
both with loving supportive
people.

Week Thirty-two: Saturday

The mother's stressful emotions reach the baby through hormonal activity and affect its behavior in the womb.

*I gladly remove
what you no longer need,
my sweet child; feel free to
relax and enjoy life.*

Week Twelve: Saturday

The placenta siphons off carbon dioxide and waste products from your baby and carries them back to its mother's blood.

*I gently exercise my body,
sweet child, while cradling
you lovingly within me.*

Week Thirty-two: Friday

Gentle exercise is good for most mothers during the last trimester of pregnancy; however, strenuous exercise shunts blood away from the uterus as muscles utilize all available oxygen, leaving less oxygen for your baby.

Darling baby,
you are developing
perfectly in every way!

Week Thirteen: Sunday

A final set of kidneys form to replace your baby's earlier more primitive set.

Sweet baby,
you are the light of our lives;
we are so grateful you are
entering our world.

Week Thirty-two: Thursday

Talking to your baby in the womb increases closeness
and enhances communication after birth.

You are growing
so big and strong,
my sweetheart; you are a
beloved child of life.

Week Thirteen: Monday

Your baby continues its rapid body growth.

As your eyesight becomes refined, little one, you are more and more aware of the beauty of your world.

Week Thirty-two: Wednesday

The pupillary light reflex appears as your baby's iris becomes capable of closing down in response to light.

*You are sweet
and healthy and strong,
little one.*

Week Thirteen: Tuesday

Cells producing the insulin hormone appear.

*You are perfect
and beautiful, little baby,
and preparing for a
wonderful life ahead.*

Week Thirty-two: Tuesday

Even with the additional fat cell accumulation, your
baby still appears quite thin.

*Your body
is strong and healthy,
my darling baby.*

Week Thirteen: Wednesday

The placenta transmits antibodies to your baby from its mother to provide immunity to certain illnesses.

*Feel the loving
warmth and protection
of your new cells,
little one.*

Week Thirty-two: Monday

Additional fat cells have accumulated under your
baby's skin.

You are such a remarkable creation of love, precious infant; I love how you are growing!

Week Thirteen: Thursday

Your baby has doubled its size in just three weeks.

*You are healthy
and strong, my darling baby,
and everyone around you
loves you very much.*

Week Thirty-two: Sunday

Your baby is now 16 inches long and weighs about
3 1/2 pounds.

Darling baby,
you are safe and
secure in your world.

Week Thirteen: Friday

The placenta blocks transmission of some infections
and drugs from the mother to the baby.

Dearest infant,
you are a powerful
individual with your own
creative intelligence.

Week Thirty-one: Saturday

Psychologists speculate that your baby's ego is
already beginning formation at this time.

*There is plenty
of room in your world
for you to grow and play,
sweet baby.*

Week Thirteen: Saturday

Hormones are produced by the placenta to maintain
the lining of the uterus and support growth of the
mother's uterus and breasts during the pregnancy.

*Precious little one,
your awareness of life is
growing and expanding
continuously.*

Week Thirty-one: Friday

Western researchers believe this time period in the
womb is the beginning of true consciousness.

Move and play,
my little sweetheart; you
are strong and perfect
in every way.

Week Fourteen: Sunday

Your baby's limbs are now fully formed, although
their movements are still undetectable by its mother.

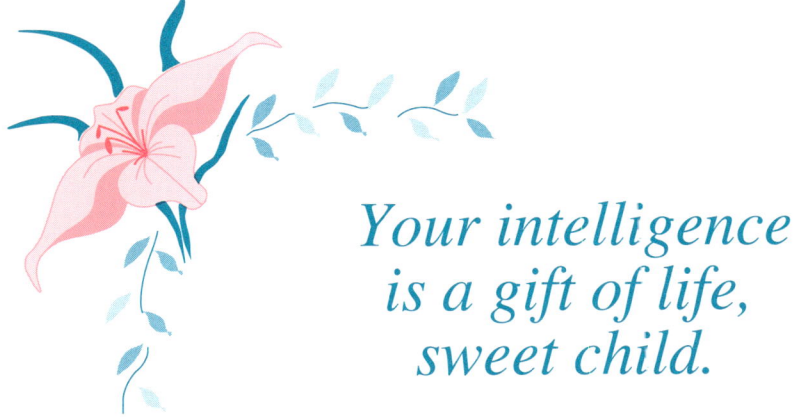

*Your intelligence
is a gift of life,
sweet child.*

Week Thirty-one: Thursday

All types of adult brain waves are now measurable in
your baby.

*Everything in
your body is working
perfectly, little baby, and I
am here to support your
precious life.*

Week Fourteen: Monday

The internal organs of your baby are fully formed but
still in need of further development to survive outside
the womb.

Precious baby,
you are continuing to
grow and develop perfectly.

Week Thirty-one: Wednesday

Growth in weight and length begins to slow down as
strength increases and refinement continues.

Darling baby,
I send you everything you
need to grow healthy
and strong.

Week Fourteen: Tuesday

Your baby is now connected to the umbilical cord.

*Everything about
you is perfect, little one;
you are a beloved child
of Life.*

Week Thirty-one: Tuesday

As your baby has been growing, the head has grown
more in proportion to the rest of its body.

Dearest baby,
you are discovering new
and exciting ways to take
in life's nourishment!

Week Fourteen: Wednesday

Swallowing and sucking begin for your baby.

Sweet child,
your intelligent mind is
gently protected until you
are ready to enter this
larger world.

Week Thirty-one: Monday

Your baby's skull is still quite delicate.

You are
growing bigger every day,
sweetheart; life supports
you in every way.

Week Fourteen: Thursday

Your baby is now three inches long.

Life is here for us
to breathe in, little one; life
supports us in our journey
of growth.

Week Thirty-one: Sunday

Your baby's lungs continue to develop but are still immature.

*You have
boundless energy,
little baby, move around
in your safe little home!*

Week Fourteen: Friday

Your baby continues its vigorous limb movements.

Darling child,
I talk to you continually to
caress you with caring
and love.

Week Thirty: Saturday

Your baby's sense of hearing is stimulated by music and singing, and gentle melodic speech, especially its mother's voice.

Your gender
is a precious part of
who you are, sweet child,
and we love whoever you
have chosen to be.

Week Fourteen: Saturday

External genitalia are now developed enough to
determine your baby's sex through ultrasound.

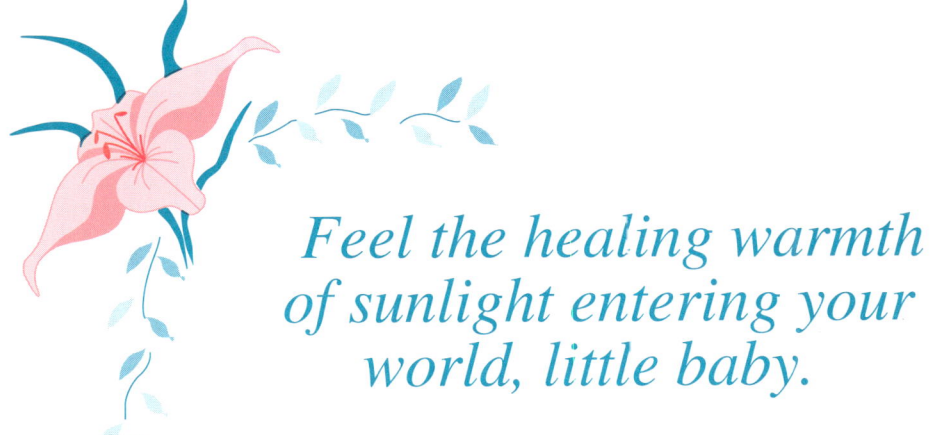

Feel the healing warmth of sunlight entering your world, little baby.

Week Thirty: Friday

Your baby's environment floods with light when you are sunbathing, stimulating its sense of sight.

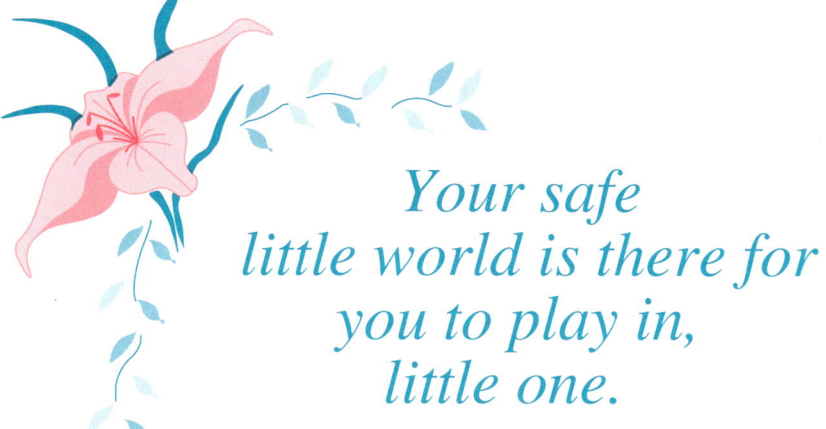

Your safe
little world is there for
you to play in,
little one.

Week Fifteen: Sunday

Your baby is moving around, although its mother
remains unaware of its movements at this time.

*Sweet little one,
can you feel our loving
caresses? We surround your
little world with love
and joy.*

Your baby's tactile senses can be stimulated by
showering and gentle abdominal massage.

You are
completely perfect
even in your tiny world,
sweet baby.

Week Fifteen: Monday

Your baby's body is developing and begins to look much like a newborn.

*Darling child,
can you sense what a
wonderful, loving world
is waiting to welcome you?*

Week Thirty: Wednesday

All of your baby's senses are now functional.

I caress
the thoughts and ideas
in your perfect little head,
sweet child.

Week Fifteen: Tuesday

Your baby's head is still relatively large in proportion to the rest of its body.

Sweet baby,
it is safe for you to take
time to grow and become
strong.

Week Thirty: Tuesday

Further development within the womb is mainly to increase your baby's size and strength.

Darling little one,
I exercise my body lovingly
and share the healthy
benefits with you.

Week Fifteen: Wednesday

When you exercise, your baby's muscles and nerves
and its sense of touch are all stimulated.

Dearest child,
I cherish this time that
you and I spend within the
same space; we are a
great team!

Week Thirty: Monday

A baby born at 30 weeks can cry weakly and breathe with difficulty; more time in the womb refines body functions in preparation for birth.

Sweet baby,
I lovingly share my
robust health and energy
with you!

Week Fifteen: Thursday

A slight increase in endorphins, the body's natural opiate, is transmitted across the placenta to your baby during light exercise.

Your world
is growing and expanding
for you, little one.

Week Thirty: Sunday

Your baby is now 14-15 inches long and weighs
about 2 1/2 to 3 pounds.

*Precious child,
you are invited to grow
and become strong and
healthy.*

Week Fifteen: Friday

Most of your baby's growth in the next few weeks is
in the torso and limb area.

*Every learning
experience is a joy,
precious child; you have
an insatiable desire to learn.*

Week Twenty-nine: Saturday

More sophisticated learning is now possible due to
nervous circuit production.

Sweet baby,
you can hold your head
high with pride! You are a
precious and beloved
child of Life.

Week Fifteen: Saturday

Your baby's head position becomes more upright,
although the head does not grow larger at this time.

You are
moving with joy and ease,
sweet baby.

Week Twenty-nine: Friday

Your baby's nervous circuits increase, making
possible increasingly refined movements.

Little baby,
you are precious and
delicate, and I will
keep you safe.

Week Sixteen: Sunday

The skin of your baby is currently thin and red.

*Your mind is
a powerful tool, little one,
for you to build a loving,
purposeful life.*

Week Twenty-nine: Thursday

Neurological functions localize to specific areas of
your baby's brain.

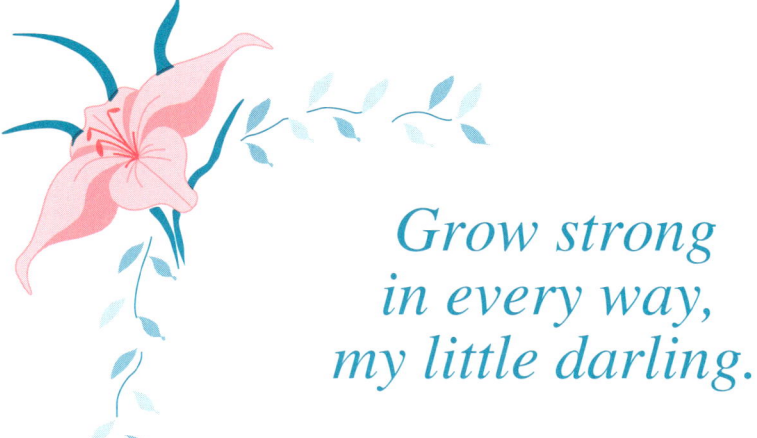

*Grow strong
in every way,
my little darling.*

Week Sixteen: Monday

Neck and back muscles are beginning to develop.

My beloved infant,
you are filled with creative
intelligence and your mind
has the power to create
wonder in your world.

Week Twenty-nine: Wednesday

Your baby's brain is growing greatly in size, surface area, and number of cells.

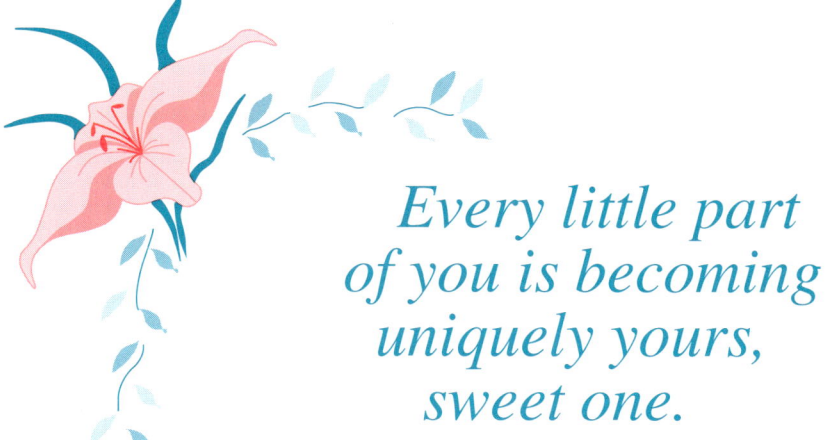

*Every little part
of you is becoming
uniquely yours,
sweet one.*

Week Sixteen: Tuesday

Ridges begin to develop in the skin on the bottom of
your baby's feet, and on the toes, hands, and fingers.

Sweet child,
you are learning to take in
nourishment and new ideas
from the world you are
entering.

Week Twenty-nine: Tuesday

Sucking and swallowing skills develop further, helping to prepare your baby for life outside the womb.

*Your bones
are strong and healthy,
little one; you are
perfectly formed.*

Week Sixteen: Wednesday

More of your baby's skeleton turns from cartilage to bone.

Listen to the beauty around you, precious baby, and communicate your joy back to the world.

Your baby continues to respond to sound, even to high frequencies that are beyond the range of adult hearing.

You are
a unique individual in
every way, and we love you
just the way you are!

Pads develop on your baby's fingertips and toes, allowing for its own individual fingerprints and footprints.

You are developing your individuality, sweet baby, and growing big and strong.

Week Twenty-nine: Sunday

Your baby's skin development continues and rapid growth is normal.

You are
growing more beautiful
each moment,
my little sweetheart!

Week Sixteen: Friday

Your baby is now approximately six inches long and weighs about three ounces.

Darling infant,
our nerves are receptive
reporters that communicate
to us with joy and ease.

Week Twenty-eight: Saturday

The development of myelin speeds up the transmission of your baby's nerve impulses.

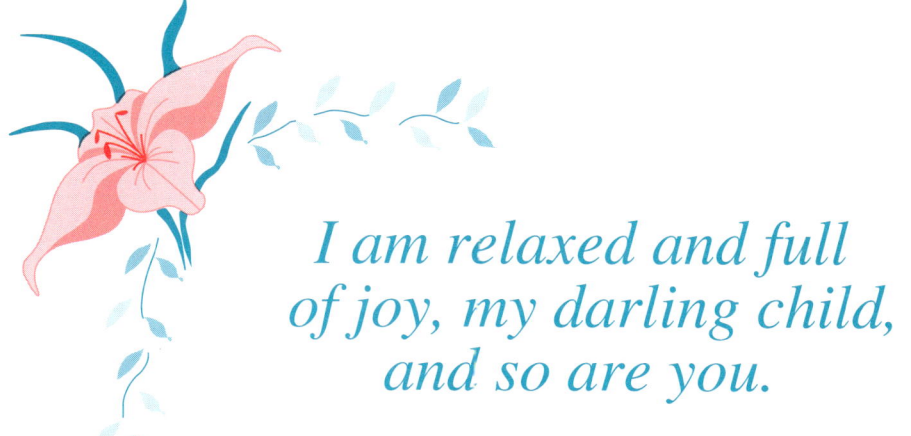

*I am relaxed and full
of joy, my darling child,
and so are you.*

Week Sixteen: Saturday

Stress reactions in the mother can cause as much as a
60% decrease in the blood flow to the uterus.

Your nervous system and your intuition will tell you much of what you need to know, little one.

Week Twenty-eight: Friday

A fatty sheath called myelin begins to develop around your baby's nerve fibers.

My loving
intelligent child, you are
developing most
beautifully!

Week Seventeen: Sunday

Your baby's head has by now become quite round.

Sweet child,
your body is learning to
communicate with itself.
We listen attentively to the
wisdom our bodies speak.

Week Twenty-eight: Thursday

Tremendous changes are taking place in your baby's nervous system.

Look around you, precious baby, and contemplate the wonder of your world.

Week Seventeen: Monday

The neck is now forming so that your baby's head can move quite easily.

Darling baby,
there is so much wonder in
the world for your senses to
experience, and I am here to
experience it with you.

Week Twenty-eight: Wednesday

At this time, your baby can actually hear, smell, and taste.

Smile, sweet child!
Use your lovely mouth
to sing and shout and take in
life's nourishment.

Week Seventeen: Tuesday

Your baby's mouth is now properly developed.

*You are able
to move through life with
joy and ease, precious child.*

Week Twenty-eight: Tuesday

Your baby is experiencing increased muscle tone.

*You are free
to look at and listen to
the wonders of your
precious world.*

Week Seventeen: Wednesday

Eyes and outer ears have become fully developed for
your baby.

*Bathe yourself
in the beauty of the light,
sweet child, and watch the
world unfold before you!*

Week Twenty-eight: Monday

Your baby's eyes are completely formed and perceive light.

*All that we want
and need, sweet child,
is cycling in and out
of our world.*

Week Seventeen: Thursday

The fetal water cycle evolves. Your baby begins to
swallow and excrete amniotic fluid.

*Your beautiful skin
protects and nourishes your
precious individuality,
my beloved child!*

Week Twenty-eight: Sunday

Your baby's skin develops fat deposits and changes
from red to its natural skin tone.

Dearest baby,
it is safe to let go of the old
and allow the new to flow
into your life.

Week Seventeen: Friday

The mother's body absorbs amniotic fluid and produces new fluid at a constant rate.

Sweet baby,
deep in your bone marrow,
you produce joy and support
and send it flowing through
your body.

Week Twenty-seven: Saturday

Your baby's red blood cell production begins shifting
entirely to the bone marrow in its own body.

Give your
little button nose a tweak
from those who love you!

Week Seventeen: Saturday

Your baby's nose is now fully developed.

*Your skin is
smooth and beautiful,
little one, and I gently
caress you with my loving
thoughts.*

Week Twenty-seven: Friday

Subcutaneous fat, called white fat, forms and fills out
the wrinkles in your baby's skin.

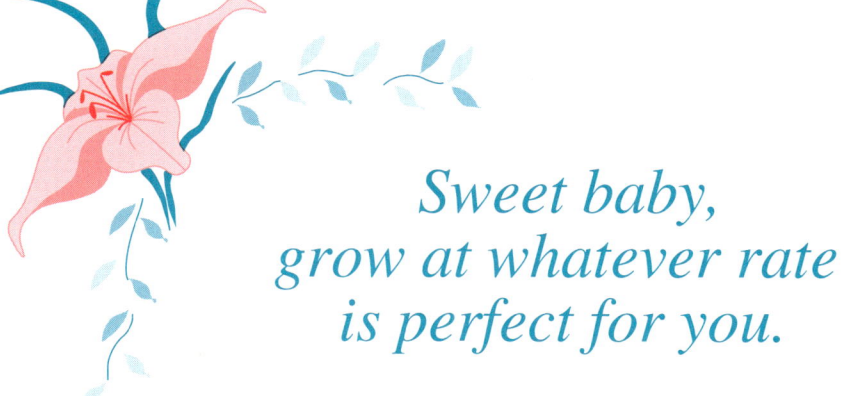

Sweet baby,
grow at whatever rate
is perfect for you.

Week Eighteen: Sunday

Developmental changes are slowing to the extent that they are described in terms of months, rather than weeks or days.

*Let the soft
down caress your back and
shoulders, dear baby, and
keep you warm and relaxed.*

Week Twenty-seven: Thursday

The downy lanugo now covers only your baby's back and shoulders.

*Sweet little
boy or girl, your gender
is a perfect expression of
who you are.*

<u>*Week Eighteen: Monday*</u>

Your baby's sexual organs are essentially formed.

*You are emerging
from your downy protection,
little one, and all is safe
in your world.*

Week Twenty-seven: Wednesday

The downy lanugo that has covered your baby's body
has begun to disappear.

Wiggle your little fingers and toes, my love, and count the blessings in your world!

Week Eighteen: Tuesday

Fingers and toes are now fully separated from their earlier weblike structure.

Infant child,
we choose to recognize
the beauty that surrounds
us in this loving world.

Week Twenty-seven: Tuesday

Your baby's eyes are now able to open and close.

My darling baby,
I cradle you inside my
tummy and celebrate
your wonderful growth.

Week Eighteen: Wednesday

Your baby is now 8-10 inches in length and weighs
6-8 ounces.

*Your beautiful eyes
are framed perfectly,
little sweetheart; you are
ready to look at your
wonderful world.*

Week Twenty-seven: Monday

The eyebrows and eyelashes of your baby have
grown and are very much in evidence.

Let the sunshine in,
sweet baby! Grow and play
in its loving warmth.

Week Eighteen: Thursday

Your baby is now sensitive to light that penetrates the
uterine wall.

Sweet child,
your hair is shiny and
healthy and an expression
of your individuality.

Week Twenty-seven: Sunday

Your baby's hair has grown longer.

Dearest baby,
it is safe to let go of all
we no longer need
in our lives.

Week Eighteen: Friday

Meconium, the early fecal matter, is beginning to collect in your baby's intestinal tract.

*Grow big and strong
and beautiful, sweet baby;
you are a precious
gift of life.*

Week Twenty-six: Saturday

Your baby is now over 12 inches long and weighs about 1 1/2 pounds.

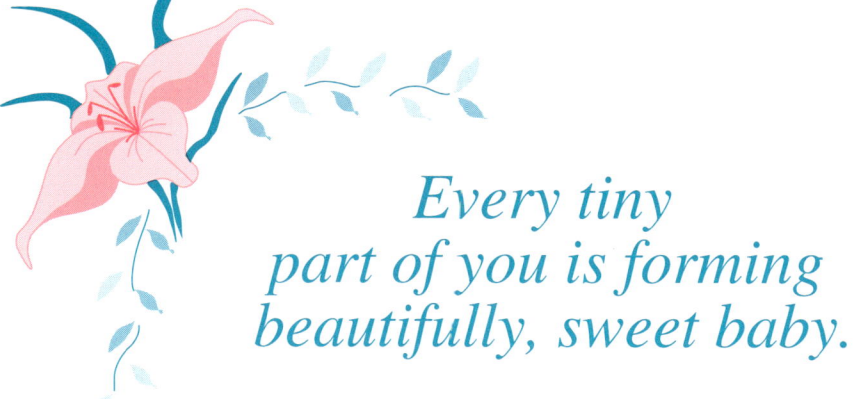

*Every tiny
part of you is forming
beautifully, sweet baby.*

Week Eighteen: Saturday

Many of your baby's deciduous teeth are well formed
under the gums.

Your lungs are forming perfectly, little one; fill your lungs with the beauty and love of life.

Week Twenty-six: Friday

Blood vessels surrounding the alveoli enable your baby to exchange oxygen and carbon dioxide after it is born.

Precious little one,
I lovingly nourish my body
and send energy and love
to you to help you grow.

Week Nineteen: Sunday

Your baby is growing rapidly at this time.

Sweet baby,
fill your lungs with the
sweetness of life.

Week Twenty-six: Thursday

For the first time, your baby has a good chance of surviving outside the womb, due to the formation of alveoli, the tiny air sacs in the lungs.

*Everything you need
to develop and grow
is coming to you perfectly,
little one.*

Week Nineteen: Monday

Lanugo, a fine downy fuzz, appears on your baby's
eyebrows and upper lip.

*Everything you need
for protection is here,
my love; you are a lovable
child of life.*

Your baby is now covered with the fuzzy down of lanugo.

You have
everything you need,
sweet baby, to be protected
and safe.

Week Nineteen: Tuesday

Eventually, lanugo will cover your baby's entire body
for the duration of the pregnancy.

*You are
increasingly capable of
breathing in the goodness
of life, dear child.*

Week Twenty-six: Tuesday

Your baby's bronchial tubes continue to branch.

*Every change
you experience is safe
and perfect for you,
my darling child.*

Week Nineteen: Wednesday

Just before birth, your baby will shed its protective
downy fuzz and replace it with hair.

Sweet baby,
you are able to release
all that you no longer need.

Week Twenty-six: Monday

The tubules of your baby's kidneys branch out.

*Your lungs
are meant to breathe in
the beauty of life,
sweet child.*

Week Nineteen: Thursday

Your baby's lungs are developing well, but are not yet mature enough to survive outside the womb.

*You are whole
and complete, and your
gender expresses your inner
self perfectly, little one.*

Week Twenty-six: Sunday

At this time your baby's ovaries or testes are completely developed.

Sweet baby,
you are invited to digest
all the wonderful ideas
life brings to you.

Week Nineteen: Friday

The digestive system of your baby has matured in development, but still needs more refinement before birth.

Dearest baby,
you are growing perfect
and healthy in every way!

Week Twenty-five: Saturday

Your baby's weight and length are increasing
steadily.

You are so beautiful, little darling! I hold you close to my heart and send you lots of love.

Week Nineteen: Saturday

Your baby's appearance is well developed.

Look at
and listen to the beauty
of your world, little one,
and cherish the memories
in your mind.

Week Twenty-five: Friday

Your baby's brain waves reflect beginning activity in
the hearing and visual systems.

*Move easily,
my little love; you are free
to move around in your
loving little world.*

Week Twenty: Sunday

Fluid has increased around your baby and it can move
and rotate in the womb with ease.

*Sweet intelligent baby,
you are creating health
and well-being with
your thoughts.*

Brain wave patterns assimilate those measured in a full-term newborn.

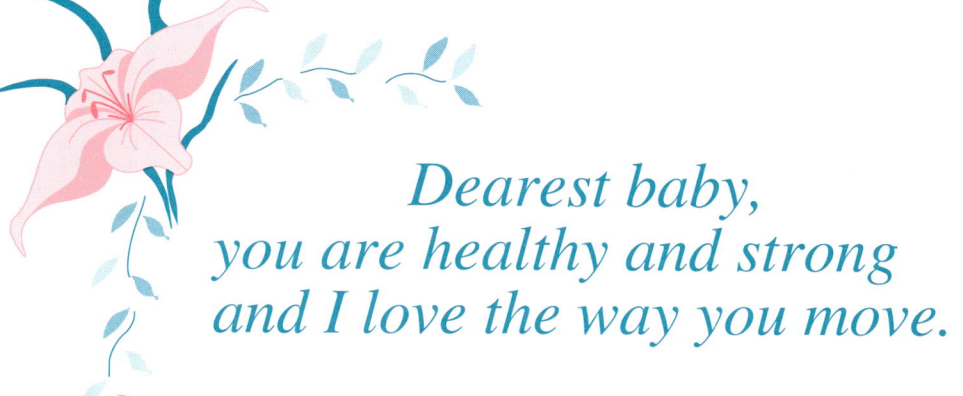

Dearest baby,
you are healthy and strong
and I love the way you move.

Week Twenty: Monday

Your baby's muscles have increased in strength.

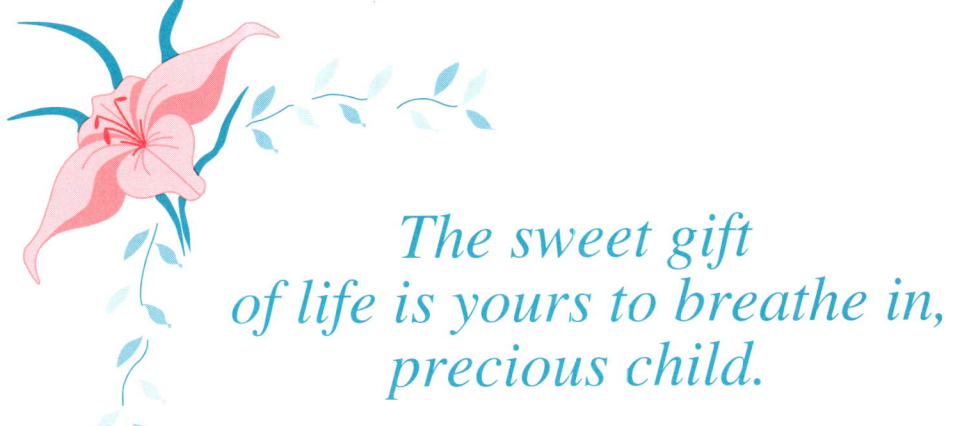

*The sweet gift
of life is yours to breathe in,
precious child.*

Week Twenty-five: Wednesday

Your baby's nostrils are opening and muscular
breathing movements begin.

Sweet little darling,
I am so full of wonder at
your movements inside me.

Week Twenty: Tuesday

Quickening, the first fetal movement felt by the mother, happens around this time.

Dearest child,
I provide for your listening
pleasure, days of pleasant
laughter, fine music, and
loving voices.

Week Twenty-five: Tuesday

External sounds such as music and voices are heard
by your baby.

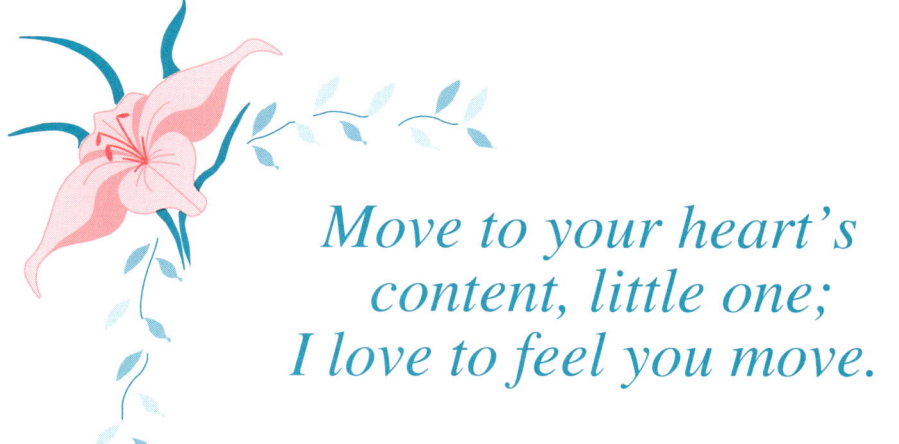

Move to your heart's
content, little one;
I love to feel you move.

Week Twenty: Wednesday

First movement feels like a bare flutter, but it continues to gain in strength each day.

Listen to the functioning of our healthy bodies, little one; we listen to our bodies and find answers to our questions about life.

Week Twenty-five: Monday

Your baby hears continuous noise from its mother's intestines and blood flow.

Darling child,
I am here to keep you
safe and warm.

Week Twenty: Thursday

Currently, your baby needs your help to maintain its body temperature.

*Your world is
filled with beautiful music,
gentle voices, and the
healing calls of nature.*

<u>*Week Twenty-five: Sunday*</u>

Your baby's inner ear is totally developed and it is
able to respond to sounds.

*Everything
you need comes to you
at the perfect time,
sweet baby.*

Week Twenty: Friday

Your baby's body still lacks a specialized fatty tissue
that produces heat.

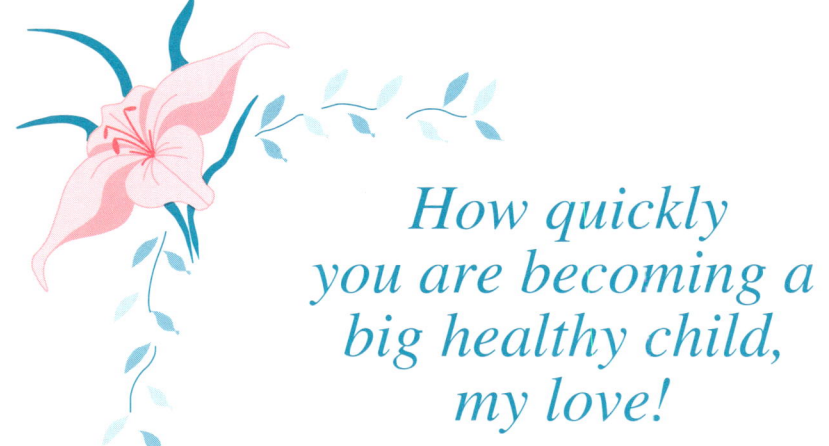

*How quickly
you are becoming a
big healthy child,
my love!*

Week Twenty-four: Saturday

General rapid growth continues through this time
period.

You are growing
so big and healthy,
little sweetheart, I love to
feel you growing inside me.

Week Twenty: Saturday

Your baby is now about 10 inches long and weighs about 12 ounces.

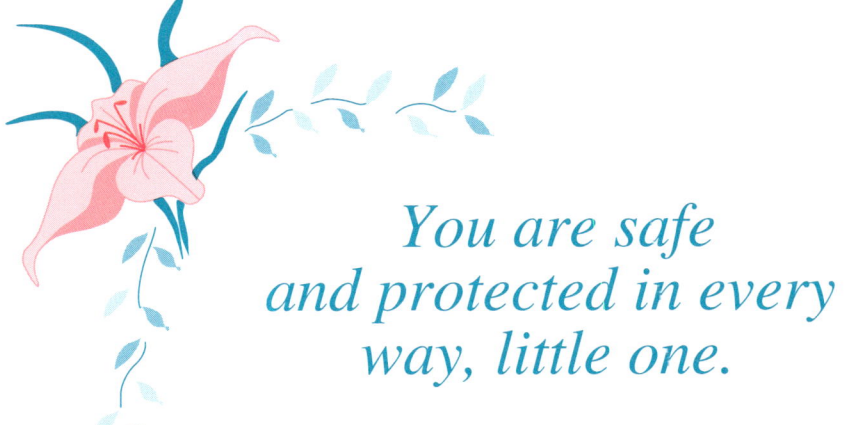

*You are safe
and protected in every
way, little one.*

Week Twenty-four: Friday

Your baby's body is now completely covered with
the creamy white vernix caseosa.

*You are warm
and secure, little one;
all is well in your world.*

Week Twenty-one: Sunday

This month, brown fat, the specialized heat-producing
fatty tissue, will begin to form in your baby's neck,
chest and crotch area.

*You are growing
into the most beautiful
little person ever,
my precious child.*

Week Twenty-four: Thursday

Your baby is now nearly 12 inches long and weighs
about one pound.

*Your skin
is smooth and beautiful,
little sweetheart, and you
are absolutely safe.*

Week Twenty-one: Monday

A creamy, white covering for your baby's skin has
begun to form.

*Sweet little baby,
every stage of your
development is a wonder!
You are perfect just
as you are.*

Week Twenty-four: Wednesday

Your baby is still lacking the characteristic "baby fat" and looks more like a very tiny old man than an infant.

*You have everything
you need, sweet baby;
you are safe and secure
and developing perfectly.*

Week Twenty-one: Tuesday

Your baby's protective cream covering, called vernix caseosa, is forming from oil gland secretions in its skin.

*Flash those
baby blues, my little love,
or will they be brown
or green?*

Week Twenty-four: Tuesday

The iris of your baby's eyes will develop pigment after birth.

*Your skin
is beautiful and perfect
for you, little one.*

Week Twenty-one: Wednesday

Vernix caseosa prevents your baby's skin from
becoming waterlogged in the amniotic fluid.

*Darling baby,
everything in the world
is yours to see and explore!*

The iris of the eye is in place.

I lovingly
care for my skin,
little sweetheart, as I know
you are caring for yours.

<u>*Week Twenty-one: Thursday*</u>

Gradually, your baby's creamy white covering will be
absorbed by the skin, but some will still be evident at
birth.

*Dearest little one,
every little detail of your
development is perfectly
taken care of; you are
beautiful!*

Week Twenty-four: Sunday

Your baby's eyebrows and eyelashes are evident.

Everything
works perfectly for you,
my sweet child.

Week Twenty-one: Friday

Most of your baby's body systems are formed and are now growing and refining themselves.

Sweet baby,
everything is here for you
to keep you healthy,
safe and loved.

The mother's body is circulating an increased blood volume to protect the baby against normal drops in maternal blood pressure.

Sweet baby,
I lovingly nourish my body
with a healthy, balanced
diet that benefits both of us.

Week Twenty-one: Saturday

A balanced maternal diet, rich in proteins and carbohydrates, helps your baby's developing organs attain normal size and cell number.

*You are growing
more perfect and beautiful
each day, little infant.*

Week Twenty-three: Friday

Your baby is now about 11 inches long.

You are welcome to express your individuality, little one, by waking and moving to your own schedule.

Week Twenty-two: Sunday

Your baby has definite sleeping and waking cycles.

*You are perfect
the way you are right now,
sweet baby. Everything
happens at the perfect time.*

Week Twenty-three: Thursday

Your baby's current leanness is due to a lack of body fat under the skin. This develops in time.

Sweet baby,
I cherish your ability to
wake and move and tell me
you are there!

Week Twenty-two: Monday

Sleeping and waking cycles are influenced by sensors in the fetus as well as by the mother's activities.

*Your blood
is full of joy circulating
to every part of you,
little one.*

Week Twenty-three: Wednesday

Your baby's red skin coloring reflects its developing
skin capillary system.

I feel your movements, little one, as I send you nourishment and love.

<u>Week Twenty-two: Tuesday</u>

Your baby generally becomes more active after its mother eats.

*You are developing
exactly as you should,
my wonderful little infant;
you are beautiful!*

Week Twenty-three: Tuesday

Currently your baby appears red, wrinkled, and lean.

Sweet baby,
you are developing new
ways to take in
life and nourishment.

Week Twenty-two: Wednesday

Your baby is now capable of strong sucking motions and can grip with its hands.

I eat a balanced, nutritious diet, my sweet baby, to nourish you as you develop.

Week Twenty-three: Monday

Good maternal nutrition is essential for this current period of brain development.

*Take a look
around you, sweetheart.
There is so much wonder
in the world to see!*

Week Twenty-two: Thursday

Your baby's eyes begin blinking movements.

My sweet intelligent child, your mind is a world of its own to explore all of life's ideas.

Week Twenty-three: Sunday

Your baby's brain is undergoing important development from now until well after birth.

*Listen to the music
of life, my little darling,
and make lots of music
of your own!*

Week Twenty-two: Friday

Bones of the ear ossify, or harden, making sound
conduction possible.

*Sweet baby,
you are growing strong
and healthy; life supports
you in every way.*

Week Twenty-two: Saturday

Your baby is about 10 1/2 inches long and weighs
about 15 ounces.

Need another calendar?

We encourage you to purchase additional *Affirmative Press* products from your local retail establishment or medical clinic. If you cannot find our products from any local sources, we will be glad to fill your order by direct mail. Please use the order form below.

Qty	Product Description	Price Each	Total
	Affirmations for your Healthy Pregnancy	$15.00	
Subtotal			
6.5% Sales Tax (if MN resident)			
Total			

Name _____

Address _____

City, State, Zip _____

Make Checks to: Affirmative Press   (612)546-9311
                 5115 Excelsior Blvd.   Suite 413
                 Minneapolis, MN 55416